THE OSTEOPOROSIS GUIDE

Best Natural Ways To Cure
Osteoporosis &
Weak Bone.

Theresa Abraham

Table Of Contents

Chapter 1

ABOUT OSTEOPOROSIS

Osteoporosis weakens bones, leaving people more prone to abrupt and unexpected fractures. The condition generally advances without any signs or discomfort and is not identified until bones shatter. You can take efforts to avoid this condition, and therapies do exist.

What is osteoporosis?

The term 'osteoporosis' means 'porous bone.' It is a condition that weakens bones, and if you have it, you are at a higher risk for abrupt and unexpected bone fractures. Osteoporosis indicates that you have diminished bone mass and strength. The condition generally develops without any signs or discomfort, and it is usually not detected until the weakening bones produce painful fractures. Most of them are fractures of the hip, wrist, and spine.

Who Gets Osteoporosis?

About 200 million individuals are thought to have osteoporosis across the globe. In the U.S., the total is roughly 54 million individuals. Although osteoporosis occurs in both men and women, women are four times more likely to get the condition than males. There are now roughly two million men in the U.S. who have osteoporosis and about 12 million more who are at risk of acquiring the disorder.

After age 50, one in two women and one in four men will have an osteoporosis-related fracture throughout their lives. Another 30% have a poor bone density which puts them at risk of developing osteoporosis. This condition is termed osteopenia.

Osteoporosis is responsible for more than two million fractures each year, and this figure continues to climb. There are things you may do to prevent osteoporosis from ever happening. Treatments may help delay the pace of bone loss if you do have osteoporosis.

What Causes Osteoporosis?
Researchers understand how osteoporosis develops even without understanding the actual explanation of why it occurs. Your bones are formed of life, developing tissue. The interior of a healthy bone appears like a sponge. This section is termed trabecular bone. An outer layer of thick bone wraps around the spongy bone. This hard shell is called cortical bone.

When osteoporosis begins, the "holes" in the "sponge" get bigger and more frequent, which weakens the interior of the bone. Bones support the body and safeguard important organs. Bones also store calcium and other minerals. When the body requires calcium, it breaks down and rebuilds bones.

This process, termed bone remodeling, feeds the body with essential calcium while keeping the bones sturdy.

Up until roughly age 30, you generally create more bone than you lose. After age 35, bone breakdown happens more quickly than bone growth, which causes a steady decrease in bone mass. If you have osteoporosis, you lose bone mass at a higher pace. After menopause, the rate of bone degradation rises significantly faster

Symptoms And Causes
What are the signs of osteoporosis?
Usually, there are no signs of osteoporosis. That is why it is often dubbed a quiet sickness. However, you should look out for the following things:
Loss of height(getting shorter by an inch or more).
Change in posture (stooping or leaning forward).

Shortness of breath (reduced lung capacity owing to squeezed disks).
Bone fractures.
Pain in the lower back.

Who is At Risk For Developing Osteoporosis?

Various risk factors raise your probability of having osteoporosis, with two of the most prominent being gender and age.
Everyone's risk for osteoporosis fractures grows with age. However, women over the age of 50 or postmenopausal women have the highest chance of getting osteoporosis. Women endure fast bone loss in the first 10 years after entering menopause, since menopause reduces the production of estrogen, a hormone that protects against excessive bone loss.

Age and osteoporosis affect guys also. You may be startled to find that males over the age of 50 are more likely to have an osteoporosis-induced bone break than to have prostate cancer. About 80,000 males each year are predicted to break a hip, and men are more likely than women to die in the year following a hip fracture.

Your chance of having osteoporosis is also tied to ethnicity. Caucasian and Asian women are more prone to acquire osteoporosis. However, African-American and Hispanic women are still in danger. African-American women are more likely than white women to die following a hip fracture.

Another aspect is bone structure and body weight. Petite and skinny persons have a higher chance of getting osteoporosis since they have less bone to lose than those with more body weight and bigger frames.

Family history also plays a function in osteoporosis risk. If your parents or grandparents have had any indicators of osteoporosis, such as a broken hip after a small fall, you may have an increased chance of acquiring the illness.

Finally, several medical problems and drugs enhance your risk. If you have or have any of the following illnesses, some of which are associated with abnormal hormone levels, you and your healthcare practitioner could consider early screening for osteoporosis.

An overactive thyroid, parathyroid, or adrenal glands.
History of bariatric (weight loss) surgery or organ transplant.
Hormone therapy for breast or prostate cancer or a history of missing periods.
Celiac disease, or inflammatory bowel disease.
Blood illnesses such as multiple myeloma.
Some drugs create negative effects that may weaken the bone and lead to osteoporosis. These include steroids, therapies for breast cancer, and drugs for managing seizures. You should chat with your healthcare

practitioner or pharmacist about the impact of your drugs on bones.

It may appear as if every risk factor is tied to something that is out of your control, but that's not true. You do have control over some of the risk factors for osteoporosis. You may address drug problems with your healthcare practitioner.

Eating habits: You are more likely to develop osteoporosis if your body doesn't have enough calcium and vitamin D. Although eating disorders like bulimia or anorexia are risk factors, they may be addressed.
Lifestyle: People who have sedentary (inactive) lives have an increased risk of osteoporosis.
Tobacco use: Smoking increases the risk of fractures.
Alcohol use: Having two drinks a day (or more) raises the risk of osteoporosis.

Diagnosis And Tests

How is osteoporosis diagnosed?
Your healthcare physician may arrange a test to offer you information about your bone health before issues occur. Bone mineral density (BMD) examinations are also known as dual-energy X-ray absorptiometry (DEXA or DXA) scans. These X-rays employ extremely tiny quantities of radiation to detect how solid the bones of the spine, hip, or wrist are. Regular X-rays will only detect osteoporosis when the illness is quite well advanced.

All women over the age of 65 should get a bone density test. The DEXA scan may be done early for women who have risk factors for osteoporosis. Men over age 70, or younger men with risk factors, should also consider undergoing a bone density test.

Management And Treatment

How is osteoporosis treated?

Treatments for established osteoporosis may include exercise, vitamin and mineral supplements, and medicines. Exercise and supplements are regularly prescribed to help you avoid osteoporosis. Weight-bearing, resistance, and balancing workouts are all vital.

What Drugs Are Used To Treat Osteporopsis?
There are various groups of drugs used to treat osteoporosis. Your healthcare practitioner will work with you to discover the greatest match. It's not realistic to declare there is one optimum medicine to treat osteoporosis. The 'best' therapy is the one that is best for you.

Prevention
How can you avoid osteoporosis?
Your food and lifestyle are two significant risk factors you may alter to avoid osteoporosis. Replacing lost estrogen with hormone treatment also offers a robust

defense against osteoporosis in postmenopausal women.

Diet

To keep strong, healthy bones, you need a diet high in calcium throughout your life. One cup of skim or 1 percent fat milk provides 300 milligrams of calcium. Besides dairy products, additional excellent sources of calcium include salmon with bones, sardines, spinach, broccoli, calcium-fortified drinks and slices of bread, dried figs, and calcium supplements. It is better to attempt to acquire calcium via food and drink.

For individuals who require supplements, remember that the body can only absorb 500 mg of calcium at a time. You should take your calcium supplements in split amounts, as anything more than 500 mg will not be absorbed.

Recommended daily allowance of calcium

Age and sex

Adults, 19-50 years

Amount 1,000 mg

Adult males, 51-70 years

Amount 1,000 mg

Adult woman, 51-70 years

Amount 1,200 mg

Adults, 71 years old and older

Amount 1,200 mg

Pregnant and breastfeeding teens

Amount 1,300 mg

Pregnant and breastfeeding adults

Amount 1,000 mg

Vitamin D is also crucial because it assists the body to absorb calcium. The recommended daily intake of vitamin D is mentioned below. Vitamin D may also be gained by sunshine exposure a few times a week or by consuming fortified milk.

Recommended daily intake of Vitamin D People by age

Infants 0-6 Months
Amount 400 IU
Infants 6-12 months
Amount 400 IU
1-3 years old
Amount 600 IU
4-8 years old
Amount 600 IU
9-70 years old
Amount 800 IU
Over 70 years old
Amount 800 IU
14-50 years old, pregnant/lactating
Amount 600 IU
Talk with your healthcare practitioner about these statistics. In rare situations, you could be recommended to take additional vitamin D. Your provider could also have ideas concerning the calcium kind; for instance, you might be urged to take calcium citrate instead of calcium carbonate. Calcium citrate does not require acid to operate, thus it may be a better alternative for persons who use antacids.

When Should You Contact The Doctor For Osteoporosis?

If you have risk factors and are worried about osteoporosis, contact your healthcare provider about getting checked, even if you are not as old as 65 (for women) or 70 (for males). Osteoporosis may be dangerous. Fractures may modify or risk your life. A considerable proportion of patients who have osteoporosis and suffer hip fractures die within one year of the fracture. Always contact your healthcare practitioner if you fall, if you are concerned about bone breakage, or if you have severe back pain that comes on quickly.

Chapter 2

BONE LIFE CYCLE

Bone tissue is continually changed by the coordinated activities of bone cells, which include bone resorption by osteoclasts and bone creation by osteoblasts, whilst osteocytes function as mechanosensory and orchestrators of the bone remodeling process. This process is under the control of local (e.g., growth factors and cytokines) and systemic (e.g., calcitonin and estrogens) factors that altogether contribute to bone homeostasis. An imbalance between bone resorption and production may result in bone disorders like osteoporosis. Recently, it has been realized that, during bone remodeling, there is extensive communication among bone cells. For instance, the linkage from bone resorption to bone creation is done via contact between osteoclasts and osteoblasts. Moreover, osteocytes create substances that regulate osteoblast and osteoclast activity, while osteocyte death is followed by osteoclastic bone resorption. The expanding information on the structure and activities of bone cells helped to a better understanding of bone biology. It has been proposed that there is a complicated connection between bone cells and other organs, suggesting the dynamic nature of bone tissue. In this review, we cover the latest facts regarding the structure and activities of bone cells and the variables that drive bone remodeling.

Bone is a mineralized connective tissue that shows four kinds of cells: osteoblasts, bone lining cells, osteocytes, and osteoclasts. Bone performs key tasks in the body, such as mobility, support, and protection of soft tissues, calcium and phosphate storage, and sheltering of bone marrow. Despite its inert look, bone is a highly dynamic organ that is continually resorbed by osteoclasts and neoformed by osteoblasts. There is evidence that osteocytes operate as mechanosensory and orchestrators of this bone remodeling process. The function of bone lining cells is not fully known, however, these cells appear to play a crucial role in tying bone resorption to bone production.

Bone remodeling is a very complicated process by which old bone is replaced by new bone, in a cycle composed of three phases:
initiation of bone resorption by osteoclasts, the transition (or reversal period) from resorption to new bone development, and the bone production by osteoblasts.

This process happens to owe to the coordinated activities of osteoclasts, osteoblasts, osteocytes, and bone lining cells which collectively create the transitory anatomical structure termed basic multicellular unit (BMU).

Normal bone remodeling is important for fracture healing and skeletal adaptation to mechanical usage, as well as for calcium homeostasis. On the other hand, an imbalance of bone resorption and production occurs in various bone disorders. For example, excessive resorption by osteoclasts without the appropriate quantity of performed bone by osteoblasts leads to bone loss and osteoporosis, while the converse may result in osteopetrosis. Thus, the balance between bone production and resorption is important and relies on the activity of various local and systemic variables including hormones, cytokines, chemokines, and biomechanical stimulation.

Recent research has demonstrated that bone regulates the activity of other organs and the bone is also impacted by other organs and systems of the body, revealing new insights and proving the complexity and dynamic nature of bone tissue.

In this review, we will examine the current evidence regarding bone cell biology, bone matrix, and the variables that impact the bone remodeling process. Moreover, we shall briefly address the impact of estrogen on bone tissue under healthy and pathological situations.

Bone Cells Osteoblasts

Osteoblasts are cuboidal cells that are situated along the bone surface constituting 4–6% of the total resident bone cells and are widely recognized for their bone-building role. These cells have morphological hallmarks of protein-producing cells, including large rough endoplasmic reticulum and conspicuous Golgi apparatus, as well as numerous secretory vesicles. As polarized cells, the osteoblasts secrete the osteoid toward the bone matrix.

Osteoblasts are generated from mesenchymal stem cells (MSC). The commitment of MSC towards the osteoprogenitor lineage needs the expression of particular genes, following timely regulated processes, including the production of bone morphogenetic proteins (BMPs) and members of the Wingless (Wnt) pathways. The expressions of Runt-related transcription factors 2, Distal-less homeobox 5, and osterix (Osx) are critical for osteoblast development. Additionally, Runx2 is a master gene of osteoblast development, as evidenced by the fact that Runx2-null animals are devoid of osteoblasts. Runx2 has been found to upregulate osteoblast-related genes such as ColIA1, ALP, BSP, BGLAP, and OCN.

Once a pool of osteoblast progenitors expressing Runx2 and ColIA1 has been created during osteoblast differentiation, there occurs a proliferation phase. In this phase, osteoblast progenitors display alkaline phosphatase (ALP) activity and are called preosteoblasts. The transition of preosteoblasts to mature osteoblasts is marked by an increase in the expression of Osx and the production of bone matrix proteins such as osteocalcin (OCN), bone sialoprotein (BSP) I/II, and collagen type I. Moreover, the osteoblasts undergo morphological modifications, becoming big and cuboidal cells.

There is evidence that additional factors such as fibroblast growth factor (FGF), microRNAs, and connexin 43 play key roles in osteoblast differentiation. FGF-2 knockout mice exhibited a lower bone mass related to an increase of adipocytes in the bone marrow, showing the role of FGFs in osteoblast development. It has also been proven that FGF-18 upregulates osteoblast differentiation in an autocrine way. MicroRNAs are involved in the control of gene expression in numerous cell types, including osteoblasts, in which certain microRNAs promote and others hinder osteoblast development. Connexin 43 is recognized to be the primary connexin in bone. The mutation in the gene encoding connexin 43 affects osteoblast development and causes skeletal deformity in mice.

The creation of bone matrix by osteoblasts happens in two basic steps: deposition of organic matrix and its subsequent mineralization. In the first stage, the osteoblasts release collagen proteins, principally type I collagen, non-collagen proteins (OCN, osteonectin, BSP II, and osteopontin), and proteoglycan including decorin and biglycan, which create the organic matrix. Thereafter, the mineralization of the bone matrix takes place in two stages: the vesicular and the fibrillar phases. The vesicular phase begins when parts with a variable diameter ranging from 30 to 200 nm, termed matrix vesicles, are released from the apical membrane domain of the osteoblasts into the freshly created bone matrix which they attach to proteoglycans and other organic components. Because of their negative charge, the sulfated proteoglycans immobilize calcium ions that are stored inside the matrix vesicles. When osteoblasts produce enzymes that break down the proteoglycans, the calcium ions are liberated from the proteoglycans and cross the calcium channels located in the matrix vesicle membrane. These channels are generated by proteins called annexins.

On the other hand, phosphate-containing compounds are destroyed by the ALP released by osteoblasts, releasing phosphate ions within the matrix vesicles. Then, the phosphate and calcium ions within the vesicles nucleate, generating the hydroxyapatite crystals. The fibrillar phase occurs when the supersaturation of calcium and phosphate ions inside the matrix vesicles leads to the rupture of these structures and the hydroxyapatite crystals spread to the surrounding matrix.

Mature osteoblasts appear as a single layer of cuboidal cells having extensive rough endoplasmic reticulum and huge Golgi complex. Some of these osteoblasts show cytoplasmic processes towards the bone matrix and reach the osteocyte processes. At this stage, the mature osteoblasts might undergo apoptosis or become osteocytes or bone-lining cells. Interestingly, round/ovoid structures including dense bodies and TUNEL-positive structures have been found within osteoblast vacuoles. These results imply that aside from professional phagocytes, osteoblasts are also able to ingest and destroy apoptotic materials during alveolar bone production.

Bone Lining Cells
Bone lining cells are quiescent flat-shaped osteoblasts that coat the bone surfaces, where neither bone resorption nor bone

creation occurs. These cells have a thin and flat nuclear profile; their cytoplasm spreads over the bone surface and reveals few cytoplasmic organelles such as profiles of rough endoplasmic reticulum and Golgi apparatus. Some of these cells display processes extending into canaliculi and gap junctions are also found between neighboring bone lining cells and between these cells and osteocytes.

The secretory activity of bone lining cells relies on the bone's physiological condition, wherein these cells might reacquire their secretory activity, boosting their size and adopting a cuboidal morphology. Bone lining cells functions are not completely understood, but it has been shown that these cells prevent the direct interaction between osteoclasts and bone matrix, when bone resorption should not occur, and also participate in osteoclast differentiation, producing osteoprotegerin (OPG) and the receptor activator of nuclear factor kappa-B ligand. Moreover, the bone lining cells, along with other bone cells, are an essential component of the BMU, an architectural structure that is present throughout the bone remodeling cycle.

Osteocytes

Osteocytes, which compose 90–95% of the total bone cells, are the most prolific and long-lived cells, with a lifetime of up to 25 years. Different from osteoblasts and osteoclasts, which have been characterized by their separate activities during bone production and bone resorption, osteocytes were originally described by their appearance and location. For decades, challenges in extracting osteocytes from the bone matrix led to the erroneous belief that these cells would be passive cells, and their roles were misread. The development of new technologies such as the discovery of osteocyte-specific markers, novel animal models, the development of procedures for bone cell separation and culture, and the construction of phenotypically stable cell lines contributed to the enhancement of the knowledge of osteocyte biology. It has been established that these cells serve various critical activities in bone.

The osteocytes are positioned inside lacunae surrounded by a mineralized bone matrix, wherein they display a dendritic shape. The shape of implanted osteocytes varies depending on the bone type. For instance, osteocytes from trabecular bone are more rounded than osteocytes from cortical bone, which have an extended shape.

Osteocytes are produced from MSCs lineage via osteoblast differentiation. In this process, four distinct phases have been proposed: osteoid-osteocyte, osteocyte, young osteocyte, and mature osteocyte. After a bone production cycle, a subset of osteoblasts becomes osteocytes integrated into the bone matrix. This process is accompanied by notable morphological and ultrastructural alterations, notably the decrease of the round osteoblast size. The number of organelles such as rough endoplasmic reticulum and Golgi apparatus decreases, and the nucleus-to-cytoplasm ratio rises, which correlates to a reduction in protein production and secretion.

During osteoblast/osteocyte transition, a cytoplasmic process begins to arise before the osteocytes have been encased into the bone matrix. The mechanisms involved in the formation of osteocyte cytoplasmic processes are not well known. However, the protein E11/gp38, also termed podoplanin may play a crucial function. E11/gp38 is significantly expressed in embedding or newly embedded osteocytes, analogous to other cell types with a dendritic shape such as podocytes, type II lung alveolar cells, and cells of the choroid plexus. It has been postulated that E11/gp38 utilizes energy from GTPase activity to interact with cytoskeletal components and molecules involved in cell motility, therefore modulating actin cytoskeleton dynamics. Accordingly, suppression of E11/gp38 expression in osteocyte-like MLO-Y4 cells has been demonstrated to prevent dendritic elongation, showing that E11/gp38 is involved in dendrite development in osteocytes.

Once the stage of mature osteocyte fully entrapped into the mineralized bone matrix is completed, numerous of the previously expressed osteoblast markers such as OCN, BSPII, collagen type I, and ALP are downregulated. On the other hand, osteocyte markers like dentine matrix protein 1 (DMP1) and sclerostin are abundantly expressed.

Bone Lining Cells

Bone lining cells are quiescent flat-shaped osteoblasts that coat the bone surfaces, where neither bone resorption nor bone creation occurs. These cells have a thin and flat nuclear profile; their cytoplasm spreads over the bone surface and reveals few cytoplasmic organelles such as profiles of rough endoplasmic reticulum and Golgi apparatus. Some of these cells display processes extending into canaliculi, and gap junctions are also found between neighboring bone lining cells and between these cells and osteocytes.

The secretory activity of bone lining cells relies on the bone physiological condition, wherein these cells might reacquire their secretory activity, boosting their size and adopting a cuboidal morphology. Bone lining cells functions are not completely understood, but it has been shown that these cells prevent the direct interaction between osteoclasts and bone matrix, when bone resorption should not occur, and also participate in osteoclast differentiation, producing osteoprotegerin (OPG) and the receptor activator of nuclear factor kappa-B ligand. Moreover, the bone lining cells, along with other bone cells, are an essential component of the BMU, an architectural structure that is present throughout the bone remodeling cycle.

Osteocytes

Osteocytes, which compose 90–95% of the total bone cells, are the most prolific and long-lived cells, with a lifetime of up to 25 years. Different from osteoblasts and osteoclasts, which have been characterized by their separate activities during bone production and bone resorption, osteocytes were originally described by their appearance and location. For decades, challenges in extracting osteocytes from the bone matrix led to the erroneous belief that these cells would be passive cells, and their roles were misread. The development of new technologies such as the discovery of osteocyte-specific markers, novel animal models, development of procedures for bone cell separation and culture, and the construction of phenotypically stable cell lines contributed to the enhancement of the knowledge of osteocyte biology. In fact, it has been established that these cells serve various critical activities in bone.

The osteocytes are positioned inside lacunae surrounded by a mineralized bone matrix, wherein they display a dendritic shape. The shape of implanted osteocytes vary depending on the bone type. For instance, osteocytes from trabecular bone are more rounded than osteocytes from cortical bone, which have an extended shape.

Osteocytes are produced from MSCs lineage via osteoblast differentiation. In this process, four distinct phases have been proposed: osteoid-osteocyte, pre osteocyte, young osteocyte, and mature osteocyte. At the conclusion of a bone production cycle, a subset of osteoblasts becomes osteocytes integrated into the bone matrix. This process is accompanied by notable morphological and ultrastructural alterations, notably the decrease of the round osteoblast size. The number of organelles such as rough endoplasmic reticulum and Golgi apparatus decreases, and the nucleus-to-cytoplasm ratio rises, which correlates to a reduction in the protein production and secretion.

During osteoblast/osteocyte transition, a cytoplasmic process begins to arise before the osteocytes have been encased into the bone matrix. The mechanisms involved in the formation of osteocyte cytoplasmic processes are not well known. However, the protein E11/gp38, also termed podoplanin may play a crucial function. E11/gp38 is significantly expressed in embedding or newly embedded osteocytes, analogous to other cell types with dendritic shape such as podocytes, type II lung alveolar cells, and cells of the choroid plexus. It has been postulated that E11/gp38 utilizes energy from GTPase activity to interact with cytoskeletal components and molecules

involved in cell motility, therefore
modulating actin cytoskeleton dynamics.
Accordingly, suppression of E11/gp38
expression in osteocyte-like MLO-Y4 cells
has been demonstrated to prevent dendritic
elongation, showing that E11/gp38 is
involved in dendrite development in
osteocytes.

Once the stage of mature osteocyte fully
entrapped into the mineralized bone matrix
is completed, numerous of the previously
expressed osteoblast markers such as OCN,
BSPII, collagen type I, and ALP are
downregulated. On the other hand,
osteocyte markers like dentine matrix
protein 1 (DMP1) and sclerostin are
abundantly expressed.

Whereas the osteocyte cell body is
positioned within the lacuna, its cytoplasmic
processes (up to 50 per each cell) traverse
small tunnels that emanate from the lacuna
space called canaliculi, producing the

osteocyte lacuno canalicular system. These cytoplasmic processes are connected to other neighboring osteocytes processes by gap junctions, as well as to cytoplasmic processes of osteoblasts and bone lining cells on the bone surface, facilitating the intercellular transport of small signaling molecules such as prostaglandins and nitric oxide among these cells. In addition, the osteocyte lacuno canalicular system is in close proximity to the vascular supply, hence oxygen and nutrients reach osteocytes, its cytoplasmic processes (up to 50 per each cell) traverse small tunnels that emanate from the lacuna space called canaliculi, producing the osteocyte lacunar canalicular system. These cytoplasmic processes are connected to other neighboring osteocytes processes by gap junctions, as well as to cytoplasmic processes of osteoblasts and bone lining cells on the bone surface, facilitating the intercellular transport of small signaling molecules such as prostaglandins and nitric oxide among these cells. In addition, the osteocyte lacunar canalicular system is close to the vascular supply, hence oxygen and nutrients reach osteocytes.

It has been calculated that the osteocyte surface is 400-fold greater than that of the entire Haversian and Volkmann systems and more than 100-fold larger than the trabecular bone surface. The cell-cell contact is also mediated by interstitial fluid that passes between the osteocytes processes and canaliculi. By the lacunar canalicular system, the osteocytes operate as mechanosensory since their linked network has the potential to sense mechanical pressures and loads, therefore facilitating the adaptation of bone to everyday mechanical stresses [55]. By this method, the osteocytes appear to operate as orchestrators of bone remodeling, via modulation of osteoblast and osteoclast activity. Moreover, osteocyte death has been identified as a chemotactic signal to osteoclastic bone resorption. In agreement, it has been shown that during bone resorption, apoptotic osteocytes are engulfed by osteoclasts.

The mechanosensitive function of osteocytes is accomplished due to the strategic location of these cells within the bone matrix. Thus, the form and spatial arrangement of the osteocytes are in harmony with their sensing and signal conveyance capabilities, enabling the translation of mechanical inputs into biochemical signals, a process that is termed the piezoelectric effect. The techniques and components by which osteocytes convert mechanical inputs to biochemical signals are not well recognized. However, two processes have been postulated. One of these is that there is a protein complex produced by a cilium and its related proteins PolyCystins 1 and 2, which has been hypothesized to be necessary for osteocyte mechanosensing and osteoblast/osteocyte-mediated bone production. The second method includes osteocyte cytoskeleton components, including focal adhesion protein complex and its numerous actin-associated proteins such as paxillin, vinculin, talin, and zyxin. Upon mechanical stimulation, osteocytes create many secondary messengers, for example, ATP, nitric oxide (NO), $Ca2+$, and prostaglandins (PGE2 and PGI2,) which regulate bone physiology. Independently of the mechanism involved, it is significant to emphasize that the mechanosensitive activity of osteocytes is feasible thanks to the complicated canalicular network, which facilitates communication among bone cells.

Osteoclasts
Osteoclasts are terminally developed multinucleated cells, which emerge from mononuclear cells of the hematopoietic stem cell lineage, under the influence of many stimuli. Among these substances, the macrophage colony-stimulating factor (M-CSF), released by osteoprogenitor

mesenchymal cells and osteoblasts, and RANK ligand, secreted by osteoblasts, osteocytes, and stromal cells, are listed. Together, these factors increase the activation of transcription factors and gene expression in osteoclasts.

Despite these osteoclastogenic variables having been well established, it has recently been proven that the osteoclastogenic potential may vary depending on the bone location studied. It has been found that osteoclasts from long bone marrow are generated quicker than in the jaw. This distinct dynamic of osteoclastogenesis probably might be attributable to the cellular makeup of the bone-site specific marrow.

During bone remodeling osteoclasts polarize; then, four kinds of osteoclast membrane domains may be observed: the sealing zone and ruffled border that are in touch with the bone matrix, as well as the basolateral and functional secretory domains, which are not in contact with the bone matrix. Polarization of osteoclasts during bone resorption includes the reorganization of the actin cytoskeleton, in which an F-actin ring that comprises a dense continuous zone of highly active podosome is created, and therefore a section of the membrane that evolves into the ruffled border is isolated. It is vital to emphasize that these domains are only produced when osteoclasts are in contact with extracellular mineralized matrix, in a process wherein $\alpha v \beta$ 3-integrin, as well as the CD44, mediates the attachment of the osteoclast podosomes to the bone surface. Ultrastructurally, the ruffled border is a membrane domain created by microvilli, which is segregated from the surrounding tissue by the clear zone, also known as the sealing zone. The clear zone is a region free of organelles found in the perimeter of the osteoclast next to the bone matrix. This sealing zone is created by an actin ring and numerous other proteins, including actin, talin, vinculin, paxillin, tensin, and actin-associated proteins including as α-actinin, fimbrin, gelsolin, and dynamin. The α v β 3-integrin binds to noncollagenous bone matrices containing-RGD sequences such as bone sialoprotein, osteopontin, and vitronectin, forming a peripheric sealing that delimits the center area, where the ruffled border is found.

The preservation of the ruffled border is also required for osteoclast activity; this structure is created because of the intensive trafficking of lysosomal and endosomal components. In the ruffled border, there is a vacuolar-type H+-ATPase (V-ATPase), which helps to acidify the resorption lacuna and hence to enable the dissolution of hydroxyapatite crystals. In this location, protons and enzymes, such as tartrate-resistant acid phosphatase (TRAP), cathepsin K, and matrix metalloproteinase-9 (MMP-9) are carried into a compartment termed Howship lacunae leading to bone disintegration. The products of this degradation are subsequently endocytosed across the ruffled border and transcytosis to the functional secretory region at the plasma membrane.

Abnormal increase in osteoclast development and activity contributes to various bone illnesses such as osteoporosis, where resorption surpasses formation causing lower bone density and increased bone fractures. In various pathologic circumstances like bone metastases and inflammatory arthritis, aberrant osteoclast activation leads to periarticular erosions and painful osteolytic lesions, respectively. In periodontitis, a disease of the periodontium induced by bacterial growth drives the migration of inflammatory cells. These cells release chemical mediators such as IL-6 and RANKL that drive the migration of osteoclasts. As a consequence, abnormally enhanced bone resorption occurs in the alveolar bone, leading to the loss of the insertions of the teeth and the advancement of periodontitis.

On the other hand, in osteopetrosis, which is a rare bone disease, genetic abnormalities that impair formation and resorption activities in osteoclasts lead to reduced bone resorption, resulting in a disproportionate increase of bone mass. These illnesses illustrate the necessity of the normal bone remodeling process for the preservation of bone homeostasis.

Furthermore, there is evidence that osteoclasts demonstrate various other activities. For example, it has been established that osteoclasts create substances termed cytokines that influence osteoblast throughout the bone remodeling cycle, which will be detailed below. Other emerging evidence suggests that osteoclasts may potentially directly govern the hematopoietic stem cell niche. These results demonstrate that osteoclasts are not just bone-resorbing cells, but also a source of cytokines that regulate the activity of other cells.

Extracellular Bone Matrix

Bone is made of inorganic salts and organic matrix. The organic matrix comprises collagenous proteins (90%), mostly type I collagen, and noncollagenous proteins like osteocalcin, osteonectin, osteopontin, fibronectin and bone sialoprotein II, bone morphogenetic proteins (BMPs), growth factors. There are other tiny leucine-rich proteoglycans including decorin, biglycan, lumican, osteo aderin, and seric proteins.

The inorganic substance of bone consists largely of phosphate and calcium ions; however, considerable quantities of bicarbonate, sodium, potassium, citrate, magnesium, carbonate, fluorite, zinc, barium, and strontium are also present.

Calcium and phosphate ions nucleate to produce the hydroxyapatite crystals, which are represented by the chemical formula $Ca_{10}(PO_4)_6(OH)_2$. Together with collagen, the noncollagenous matrix proteins create a scaffold for hydroxyapatite deposition and such interaction is responsible for the characteristic stiffness and resistance of bone tissue.

The bone matrix forms a sophisticated and ordered framework that offers mechanical support and plays a crucial function in bone homeostasis. The bone matrix may release many chemicals that interfere with the bone cell's activity and, accordingly, has a role in bone remodeling. Once loss of bone mass alone is inadequate to generate bone fractures, it is proposed that additional variables, particularly changes in the bone matrix proteins and their alterations, are of critical relevance to the understanding and prediction of bone fractures. It is recognized that collagen plays a key role in the construction and function of bone tissue.

Accordingly, it has been proven that there is a fluctuation in the concentration of bone matrix proteins with age, diet, illness, and antiosteoporotic therapy which may contribute to post-yield deformation and fracture of the bone. For instance, in vivo, and in vitro studies have indicated that the increase in hyaluronic acid synthesis following parathyroid hormone (PTH) administration was connected to subsequent bone resorption indicating a probable linkage between hyaluronic acid production and the increase in osteoclast activity.

Interactions between Bone Cells and Bone Matrix

As previously noted, bone matrix not only provides support for bone cells but also plays a critical function in controlling the activity of bone cells via various adhesion molecules. Integrins are the most frequent adhesion molecules involved in the contact between bone cells and bone matrix. Osteoblasts create contacts with bone matrix using integrins, which identify and bind to RGD and other sequences found in bone matrix proteins including osteopontin, fibronectin, collagen, osteopontin, and bone sialoprotein. The most prevalent integrins found in osteoblasts are $\alpha 1 \beta 1$, $\alpha 2 \beta 1$, and $\alpha 5 \beta$. These proteins also play a crucial role in osteoblast organization on the bone surface during osteoid formation.

On the other hand, the interaction between osteoclasts and the bone matrix is crucial for osteoclast activity, as previously indicated, bone resorption occurs only when osteoclasts connect to the mineralized bone surface. Thus, during bone resorption, osteoclasts express $\alpha v \beta 3$ and $\alpha 2 \beta 1$ integrins to interact with the extracellular matrix, in which the former bind to bone-enriched RGD-containing proteins, such as bone sialoprotein and osteopontin, while β 1 integrins attach to collagen fibrils. Despite these attachments, osteoclasts are very motile even with active resorption and, as migratory cells, osteoclasts do not express cadherins. However, it has been proven that cadherins allow close interaction between osteoclast precursors and stromal cells, which produce critical growth factors for osteoclast formation.

Integrins perform a moderating function in osteocyte-bone matrix interactions. These interactions are necessary for the mechanosensitive function of these cells, wherein signals triggered by tissue deformation are created and amplified. It is still not known which integrins are involved, however, it has been reported that β 3 and β 1 integrins are involved in osteocyte-bone matrix contact. These interactions occur between the osteocyte body and the bone matrix of the lacuna wall as well as between canalicular walls and the osteocyte processes.

Only a tiny pericellular gap filled by a fluid separates the osteocyte cell body and processes from a mineralized bone matrix. The gap between the osteocyte cell body and the lacunar wall is typically 0.5–1.0 µm broad, but the distance between the membranes of osteocyte processes and the canalicular wall ranges from 50 to 100 nm. The chemical composition of the pericellular fluid has not been properly determined. However, a broad array of macromolecules generated by osteocytes such as osteopontin, osteocalcin, dentin matrix protein, proteoglycans, and hyaluronic acid is present.

The osteocytes and their processes are surrounded by a non-organized pericellular matrix; fragile fiber connections were identified inside the canalicular network, nicknamed "tethers". It has been postulated that perlecan is a potential compound of these tethers. Osteocyte processes may also connect directly via the "hillocks," which are projecting structures coming from the canalicular walls. These structures create tight interactions, probably utilizing β 3-integrins, with the membrane of osteocyte processes. Thus, these structures appear to play a major part in the mechanosensitive function of osteocytes, by detecting the fluid flow movements together with the pericellular space, triggered by mechanical load forces. In addition, the fluid flow movement is also necessary for the bidirectional solute transport in the pericellular space, which modulates osteocyte signaling pathways and communication among bone cells.

Local and Systemic Factors That Regulate Bone Homeostasis

Bone remodeling is a very complicated cycle that is performed by the cooperative activities of osteoblasts, osteocytes, osteoclasts, and bone lining cells. The creation, proliferation, differentiation, and activity of these cells are governed by local and systemic stimuli. The local factors comprise autocrine and paracrine molecules such as growth factors, cytokines, and prostaglandins generated by the bone cells alongside components of the bone matrix that are released during bone resorption. The systemic factors which are critical to the maintenance of bone homeostasis include parathyroid hormone (PTH), calcitonin, 1,25-dihydroxyvitamin D3 (calcitriol), glucocorticoids, androgens, and estrogens. Similar to PTH, PTH-related protein (PTHrP), which likewise binds to the PTH receptor, has also been demonstrated to promote bone remodeling.

Estrogen performs critical functions for bone tissue homeostasis; the reduction in estrogen levels during menopause is the major cause of bone loss and osteoporosis. The methods by which estrogen affects bone tissue are not known. Nevertheless, multiple investigations have indicated that estrogen preserves bone homeostasis by suppressing osteoblast and osteocyte death and avoiding excessive bone resorption. The estrogen reduces osteoclast production and activity as well as causes osteoclast apoptosis. It has been postulated that estrogen inhibits osteoclast development by decreasing the creation of the osteoclastogenic cytokine RANKL by osteoblasts and osteocytes. Moreover, estrogen induces these bone cells to generate osteoprotegerin (OPG), a decoy receptor of RANK in osteoclast, thereby suppressing osteoclastogenesis. In addition, estrogen reduces osteoclast formation by lowering the levels of other osteoclastogenic cytokines such as IL-1, IL-6, IL-11, TNF-α, TNF-β, and M-CSF.

Estrogen works directly on bone cells through its estrogen receptors α and β found on these cells. Moreover, it has been established that osteoclast is a direct target for estrogen. Accordingly, immunoexpression of estrogen receptor β has been observed in alveolar bone cells of estradiol-treated female rats. Moreover, the increased immunoexpression found in TUNEL-positive osteoclasts demonstrates that estrogen contributes to the regulation of osteoclast lifespan directly through estrogen receptors. These results highlight the relevance of estrogen for the maintenance of bone homeostasis.

Bone Remodeling Process
The bone remodeling cycle takes place inside bone cavities that need to be reshaped. In these cavities, there is the formation of temporary anatomical structures called basic multicellular units (BMUs), which are comprised of a group of osteoclasts ahead forming the cutting cone and a group of osteoblasts behind forming the closing cone, associated with blood vessels and the peripheral innervation. It has been postulated that BMI is covered by a canopy of cells (perhaps bone lining cells) that constitute the bone remodeling

compartment(BRC). The BRC appears to be related to bone lining cells on the bone surface, which in turn are in contact with osteocytes encased inside the bone matrix.

The bone remodeling cycle starts with an initiation phase, which consists of bone resorption by osteoclasts, followed by a period of bone creation by osteoblasts but between these two phases, there is a transition (or reversal) phase. The cycle is completed by coordinated activities of osteocytes and bone lining cells. In the initiation phase, under the action of osteoclastogenic factors like RANKL and M-CSF, hematopoietic stem cells are recruited to particular bone surface regions and develop into mature osteoclasts that commence bone resorption.

It is known that during the bone remodeling cycle, there are direct and indirect communications among bone cells in a process termed coupling mechanism, which comprises soluble coupling components held in the bone matrix that would be released following osteoclast bone resorption. For instance, substances such as insulin-like growth factors (IGFs), transforming growth factor β (TGF-β), BMPs, FGF, and platelet-derived growth factor (PDGF) tend to operate as coupling factors, as they are held in bone matrix and released during bone resorption. This concept is supported by genetic research in people and animals as well as by pharmacological investigations.

Recently, it has been reported that another family of molecules termed semaphorins is involved in bone cell communication during bone remodeling. During the early phase, osteoblast development and activity must be suppressed, to eliminate the damaged or old bone. The osteoclasts express a protein called semaphorin4D (Sema4D) that suppresses bone growth during bone resorption. Semaphorins comprise a large family of glycoproteins which are not only membrane-bound but also exist as soluble forms that are found in a wide range of tissues and shown to be involved in diverse biological processes such as immune response, organogenesis, cardiovascular development, and tumor progression. In bone, it has been postulated that semaphorins are also engaged in cell-cell communication between osteoclasts and osteoblasts throughout the bone remodeling cycle.

Sema4D produced in osteoclasts interacts with its receptor (Plexin-B1) present in osteoblasts and suppresses the IGF-1 pathway, important for osteoblast development, indicating that osteoclasts restrict bone production by producing Sema4D. Conversely, another member of the semaphorin family (Sema3A) has been discovered in osteoblasts and is considered an inhibitor of osteoclastogenesis. Thus, throughout the bone remodeling cycle, osteoclasts block bone creation by expressing Sema4D, to commence bone resorption, while osteoblasts produce Sema3A that inhibits bone resorption, before bone synthesis.

Recent studies also reveal the presence of additional variables engaged in the coupling process throughout the bone remodeling cycle. One of these factors is ephrinB2, a membrane-bound protein produced in mature osteoclasts, which binds to ephrinB4, present in the plasma membrane of osteoblasts. The ephrinB2/ephrinB4 binding transduces bidirectional signals, which promote osteoblast development, while the opposite signaling (ephrinB4/ephrinB2) suppresses osteoclastogenesis. These results imply that the ephrinB2/ephrinB4 pathway may be implicated in the stopping of bone resorption and triggering osteoblast development in the transition period.

In addition, it has been revealed that ephrinB2 is also expressed in osteoblasts. Furthermore, mature osteoclasts release a variety of substances that drive osteoblast development such as the secreted signaling molecules Wnt10b, BMP6, and the signaling sphingolipid, sphingosine-1-phosphate. These results reveal a very complicated mechanism of ephrins and the involvement of additional variables in osteoclast/osteoblast communication throughout the bone remodeling cycle. On the other hand, despite the research revealing the role of semaphorins and ephrins on osteoclast/osteoblast communication, the direct interaction between mature osteoblasts and osteoclasts has not been established in vivo and it is still contentious.

Besides osteoclasts and osteoblasts, it has been proven that osteocytes play significant functions throughout the bone remodeling cycle. In reality, under the influence of various circumstances, the osteocytes operate as orchestrators of the bone remodeling process, creating substances that impact osteoblast and osteoclast activity. For example, mechanical stress induces osteocytes to create substances that exert an anabolic effect on the bone such as PGE2, prostacyclin (PGI2), NO, and IGF-1. On the other hand, mechanical unloading downregulates anabolic hormones and promotes osteocytes to generate sclerostin and DKK-1, which are inhibitors of osteoblast activity, as well as specific factors that drive local osteoclastogenesis. Sclerostin is a product of the SOST gene and is known to be a negative regulator of bone formation, by antagonizing in osteoblasts the activities of Lrp5, a major receptor of the Wnt/β-catenin signaling cascade.

Osteocyte apoptosis has been demonstrated to operate as a chemotactic signal for local osteoclast recruitment. Accordingly, it has been shown that osteoclasts swallow apoptotic osteocytes, indicating that osteoclasts can remove dead osteocytes and/or osteoblasts from a remodeling region. Moreover, it is stated that the osteoclastogenic factors are also generated by live osteocytes closing the dying osteocytes. There is evidence that osteocytes operate as the major source of RANKL to stimulate osteoclastogenesis, however, this factor has also been found to be generated by other cell types such as stromal cells, osteoblasts, and fibroblasts.

Thus, there are still questions concerning the specific osteoclastogenesis-stimulating substances released by osteocytes. Recent studies have focused on certain substances that may be possibilities for signaling between osteocyte death and osteoclastogenesis. For instance, in bones exposed to fatigue loading, surviving osteocytes adjacent to the apoptotic one's display, despite high RANKL/OPG ratio, elevated levels of vascular endothelial growth factor (VEGF) and monocyte chemoattractant protein-1 (CCL2) encouraging an increase in local osteoclastogenesis. It has been postulated that osteocytes operate as the major source of RANKL to stimulate osteoclastogenesis. In addition, an increase in RANKL/OPG ratio produced by osteocytes was also detected in connexin43-deficient rats, indicating that a breakdown in cell-to-cell contact between osteocytes may trigger the production of local pro osteoclastogenic cytokines. High mobility group box protein 1 (HMGB1) and M-CSF have also been hypothesized to be generated by osteocytes that drive osteoclast recruitment during bone remodeling. Thus, more research is necessary to address this problem.

Endocrine Functions of Bone Tissue
The traditional roles of bone tissue, besides mobility, are support and protection of soft tissues, calcium, and phosphate storage, and sheltering of bone marrow. Additionally,

recent research has focused on the bone endocrine capabilities which can impact other organs. For instance, osteocalcin generated by osteoblasts has been found to behave in other organs. Osteocalcin may be found in two distinct forms: carboxylated and undercarboxylated. The carboxylated form has a significant affinity to the hydroxyapatite crystals, persisting inside the bone matrix after its mineralization. The undercarboxylated form exhibits decreased attraction to minerals, owing to the acidity of the bone matrix during osteoclast bone resorption, and subsequently, it is carried by the circulation, reaching other organs. It has been established that undercarboxylated osteocalcin has certain effects on the pancreas, adipose tissue, testis, and the neurological system. In the pancreas, osteocalcin works as a positive regulator of pancreatic insulin secretion and sensitivity as well as for the proliferation of pancreatic β-cells. In the adipose tissue, osteocalcin promotes adiponectin gene expression which in turn improves insulin sensitivity. In the testis, osteocalcin may bind to a particular receptor in Leydig cells and improves testosterone production and, thus, increases fertility. Osteocalcin also enhances the production of monoamine neurotransmitters in the hippocampus and inhibits gamma-aminobutyric acid (GABA) synthesis, boosting learning and memory abilities.

Another endocrine function of bone tissue is encouraged by osteocytes. These cells can control phosphate metabolism through the synthesis of FGF23, which operates on other organs such as the parathyroid gland and kidneys to lower the circulating levels of phosphates. Osteocytes also operate on the immune system by changing the milieu in primary lymphoid organs and consequently regulating lymphopoiesis. Not only osteocytes but also osteoblast and osteoclast activities are recognized to impact the immune system, especially upon bone inflammatory destruction. Indeed, the finding of communicative interaction between skeletal and immune systems led to a new branch of research termed osteoimmunology.

Conclusions

The study of the structural, molecular, and functional biology of bone is vital for the better appreciation of this tissue as a multicellular unit and a dynamic structure that can also work as an endocrine tissue, a role yet little understood. In vitro and in vivo research have proven that bone cells react to numerous stimuli and chemicals, adding to the improved knowledge of bone cell plasticity. Additionally, bone matrix integrins-dependent bone cell interactions are crucial for bone production and resorption. Studies have addressed the role of the lacunar canalicular system and the pericellular fluid, via which osteocytes operate as mechanosensory, for the adaptation of bone to mechanical stresses.

Hormones, cytokines, and factors that affect bone cell activity, such as sclerostin, ephrinB2, and semaphoring, have played a vital role in bone histophysiology under normal and pathological situations. Thus, such a greater knowledge of the dynamic structure of bone tissue will undoubtedly assist to manage novel treatment approaches to bone illnesses.

Chapter 3

LIVING WITH OSTEOPOROSIS

What can you do if you are living with osteoporosis?

If you have osteoporosis, you should continue with the lifestyle steps outlined previously in terms of eating healthily, getting adequate exercise, avoiding excessive caffeine and alcohol intake, and not smoking. Make sure that you follow the instructions of your healthcare practitioner. You should do everything that you can to avoid falls inside and outside of your house. You may wish to start with a medical assessment, which might lead to your healthcare professional giving assistive equipment.

Living with osteoporosis doesn't need to be daunting and it doesn't imply that your life can't be as full as it was before. Starting a healthy bone lifestyle may help you manage osteoporosis in your everyday life. Follow these strategies given by other patients with osteoporosis. They will allow you to take charge of your everyday life as well as help strengthen your bones and lessen the chance of fractures.

Self Care

Taking proactive involvement in osteoporosis therapy is vital. Getting more exercise, eating a balanced diet rich in calcium and vitamin D, and decreasing bad behaviors like smoking or excessive drinking can assist to preserve bone health.

Don't smoke

People who smoke have a larger risk of fracture than nonsmokers and require a longer time to recover. Women who smoke frequently generate less estrogen and are likely to enter menopause sooner, which may contribute to greater bone loss. Calcium absorption is also lower in smokers.

Drink alcohol in moderation
People who consume significant quantities of alcohol have an increased chance of getting osteoporosis. They have less bone mass and lose bone more rapidly due to alcohol's influence on bone. Drinking may also raise the likelihood of falling and fracturing a bone. Experts advocate consuming no more than two alcoholic drinks every day. One alcoholic drink is equivalent to 12 ounces of beer, 5 ounces of wine, or 1½ ounces of liquor.

Stay active
Exercise or other physical activity that builds bones may help preserve bone mass. Weight-bearing and resistance activities are highly effective. Flexibility and balance exercises assist to prevent falls and minimize fracture risk. To receive the health advantages of exercise, undertake weight-bearing and resistive exercise for 30 minutes every day, five days a week. It's normal to work out for 10 or 15 minutes at a

time then take a rest and later finish. Check with a doctor before beginning an exercise regimen.

Get the right quantity of calcium and vitamin D.
Calcium intake is essential to prevent bone loss. How much calcium a person requires varies on gender, age, and risk for osteoporosis. The greatest supply of calcium comes from foods such as dairy products, black-eyed peas, or calcium-fortified non-dairy products.

Women and men aged 19 to 49 and pregnant or breastfeeding women require 1,000 milligrams (mg) of calcium per day. Individuals on corticosteroids, postmenopausal women who aren't taking estrogen supplements, and women and men aged 50 and older require 1,200 mg per day. Those who cannot consume dairy or calcium-enriched meals could select calcium supplements.

Vitamin D boosts the amount of calcium the body absorbs from diets. Some persons may obtain adequate vitamin D by exposing the face, arms, and hands to noon sunshine for 10 to 15 minutes, two or three days a week. Other effective sources of vitamin D include liver, fish oil, vitamin D-fortified meals, and Vitamin D3 supplements

Take your osteoporosis prescription and be sure to attend all your monthly visits.
It is crucial to remember that osteoporosis is a chronic illness. To maintain preserving your bones and minimize your risk of fracture your prescription may need to be taken for many years. It is crucial to take your medicine as advised by your doctor, and don't stop taking it even if you feel well. Attend the regular visits arranged by your doctor and be sure to get bone scans and any other tests that are advised to monitor your therapy and assess your bone health.

Seek help
Talk to your doctor and healthcare team –
your pharmacist, dietician, physiotherapist,
occupational therapist, and specialist can
advise you about your lifestyle habits, diet,
and exercise to help you live with
osteoporosis.

Feed your bones
Eat a healthy, balanced diet with enough
calcium and vitamin D
Watch your diet and learn which foods are
rich in calcium and vitamin D – these
important minerals work together to keep
your bone strong. Aim to eat a varied and
healthy range of foods – lots of fresh fruit
and vegetables, meats and fish, and dairy
products are the essential ingredients for
strong healthy bones.

Maintain a healthy weight
When you have osteoporosis, being under or
overweight can interfere with your bone
health and increase your risk of fractures.

Talk to your doctor or nutritionist who can help with some tips to get your weight in a healthy range.

Be careful when bending, twisting, and lifting
Some patients find that they can't bend in the same way they could before they had osteoporosis. So be careful when doing household chores – space out your activities during the day or week, you don't need to do them all at once. And ask for help to lift and carry things if you need to.

Build stronger bones with exercise
Regular weight-bearing exercises and muscle-strengthening exercise is a great way to build stronger bones and help protect against future fractures.
3 Walking is beneficial for osteoporosis too, so if you can, try to walk to work or the shops - every little bit helps.

Take caution while out and about

People with osteoporosis might sometimes feel terrified of falling, particularly when outside their home surroundings. On public transit, don't be hesitant to ask for a seat, particularly if it is packed. And take caution while getting on and off public transit and out of vehicles and taxis.

Avoid consuming too much alcohol
Heavy drinking may inhibit bone growth. It may also raise your chance of falling and fracturing a bone.

Quit smoking
We all know that cigarettes are terrible for your health. But did you know that cigarettes also make it tougher for your bones to absorb calcium? Smoking raises the risk of hip fracture by up to 1.8 times. If you can avoid smoking, you should.

Get plenty of rest

Poor sleep has been found to impede your body's capacity to manufacture new bones, resulting in more brittle bones.
6 Try to obtain at least 7–9 hours of sleep every night.

Prevent falls within your home
Keep your flooring clean of clutter, including throw rugs and unsecured cables and cords. Use only non-skid goods if you have mats, carpets, or area rugs.
Make sure your lighting is bright enough so that you can see clearly.
Do not use cleansers that make your flooring slippery.
Clean up any spills that occur quickly.
Use grab bars in the bathroom and handrails on stairways.

Prevent falls outside your home
Make sure illumination is sufficient in all locations outside your house.
Use a backpack or other form of bag that leaves your hands free.

Keep places outdoors in excellent shape and clear of clutter.

Wear sensible shoes with non-slip soles.

This is by no means a full list of things that you can do to assist avoid falls, but this is a starting point. Also, remember to take your time. You could be less cautious if you are in a rush.

Remember that you can enjoy an active and satisfying life even if you do have osteoporosis. You and your healthcare practitioner can work together to make this happen.

Chapter 4

**BEST NATURAL WAYS TO
TREAT/PREVENT OSTEOPOROSIS**

1. Olive Oil, Dates, Cheese, and Honey:
Make a paste with one teaspoon of olive oil,
2-3 dates, 2 tablespoons of cheese, and one
teaspoon of honey. Apply this on bread and
it to girls once a week from an early age to
protect them from osteoporosis naturally.

2. Sesame Seeds: Boil one 1-2 tablespoon
crushed sesame seeds in 1 glass of milk and
drink it every day before going to bed. Zinc,
Iron, Phosphorus, Magnesium, Fiber, and
Calcium in Sesame seeds are ideal to cure
osteoporosis.

3. Bovine Colostrum Milk or Cheese: Bovine
Colostrum cheese provides protein, carbs,
lipids, vitamins, and minerals. The best
protein in it is 100 times better than cow's

milk. It has been demonstrated that colostrum milk or cheese boosts growth hormones in circulation.
Bovine Colostrum also carries hormones in it or chemicals that encourage " fresh bone formation". Take 5-8 teaspoons every day for one week then twice a week and continue for 2 or 3 months for strong and healthy bones.

4. Milk Butter(Lassi): Mixtures of these natural foods are the greatest natural, simple and quick solution to treat bone from osteoporosis and make bone healthy and strong. Low-fat milk and yogurt are rich in lactose and sugar, which are incredibly helpful for bone health. You may take vitamin D from the diet by consuming one cup every day for breakfast.

5. Blackstrap Molasses: Molasses includes a variety of vital minerals such as calcium, magnesium, manganese, potassium, copper, iron, phosphorus, chromium, cobalt, and

sodium. Calcium is the cornerstone for strong and healthy bones but magnesium is vital for bones.

Blackstrap molasses include both of these. It defends the body from bone disorders. We suggest 2 teaspoons twice a day to create healthy and stronger bones. With the suggested dosage you also complete your daily need of vitamins and minerals and also the ideal tonic to restore prior deficits.

6. Coconut water: Coconut water is the finest natural source of vitamins and minerals including calcium, magnesium, phosphorus, salt, sulfur, and chlorine. Also, enhance the immune system naturally and quickly.

Inorganic acids in coconut water have a vital function in bone development. Continued usage of one cup of coconut water for two weeks to three months is the finest natural and easiest technique to get rid of osteoporosis or weak bones.

7. Water Chestnut and Colchicum Luteum:
Make a fine powder using an equal amount
of water chestnut and Colchicum luteum.
Keep in a bottle and every day consume one
tablespoon with one glass of milk two times
a day to obtain stronger bones naturally.

8. Green Leafy Veggies: Fresh green
vegetables are also the finest way to acquire
vitamin D naturally. Add every day to your
eating plan.

9. Citrus Fruits: Fresh fruit juice like orange,
pineapple, lime, and lemon offers very many
key elements to strengthen bone density.
Vitamin C in these fruits is the finest source
to preserve bone strength.

10. Omega-3: Salmon, sardines, tuna, and
eggs are the greatest natural source of
Omega-3 and vitamin D which is very much
essential for strong Bones.

11. Almond and Figs: Almond and Figs milk every day for two-three months is the greatest natural option to get rid of this condition quickly. Just soak 6-7 almonds and 2-3 figs in one glass of milk overnight and the following morning peel off the almond and mix it. You may add 1 teaspoon of honey.

12. Fennel Seeds: elements like calcium, phosphorus, and magnesium in fennel seeds aid to improve the strength and growth of bones. Fennel seeds can slow down the formation of cells that degrade bone and cause osteoporosis. Daily chewing 1 teaspoon of fennel seeds for two months makes bone strong.

Best Exercise For Osteoporosis
It's never too late to start a bone-healthy fitness regimen, even if you already have osteoporosis.

You may fear that being active means you're more prone to fall and break a bone. But the contrary is true. A regular, carefully organized fitness program may help reduce falls and fractures. That's because exercise strengthens bones and muscles and improves balance, coordination, and flexibility. That's crucial for persons with osteoporosis.

Check With Your Doctor
Before you start a new fitness plan, check with your doctor and physical therapist. They can tell you what's safe for your stage of osteoporosis, your exercise level, and your overall health.

There is no one fitness strategy that's optimal for everyone with osteoporosis. The regimen you pick should be unique to you and based on your:
Fracture risk
Muscle strength
Range of motion

84

Level of physical activity

Fitness

Gait Balance

Your doctor also will evaluate any other health conditions that have a bearing on your capacity to exercise, such as obesity, high blood pressure, and heart disease. They may recommend you to a specialist-trained physical therapist who may teach you exercises that concentrate on body mechanics and posture, balance, resistance weights, and other approaches.

Weight-Bearing Exercises for Osteoporosis

Don't let the name mislead you — these sorts of exercises aren't about pumping iron. They are exercises you undertake on your feet so that your bones and muscles have to struggle against gravity to keep you standing. Your bones respond to their weight by growing up and becoming stronger.

There are two forms of weight-bearing exercise: high-impact and low-impact. High-impact involves routines like:
Jogging
Jumping rope
Step aerobics
Tennis or other racquet sports
Yard labor, such as pulling a lawnmower or heavy gardening
Moderate impact workouts may include:
Climbing stairs
Dancing
Hiking
But be cautious. If your osteoporosis is severe, high-impact weight-bearing workouts may not be safe for you. Talk to your doctor about your exercise program. They may propose that you concentrate on low-impact workouts that are less prone to cause fractures and yet build up your bone density. These include:
Elliptical training machines
Low-impact aerobics
Stair-step machines

Walking (either outdoors or on a treadmill machine).

If you're new to exercise or haven't worked out for a long time, you should aim to progressively increase the quantity you do until you reach 30 minutes of weight-bearing activity per day on most days of the week.

Strengthen Your Muscles

Working your muscles is important because it may help reduce fall-related fractures. Functional strength and balance exercises should be part of your program.

These workouts may involve simple actions like standing and rising on your toes, raising your body weight with exercises like push-ups or squats, and utilizing equipment such as:

Elastic exercise bands

Free weights

Weight machines

Add strength-training routines to your workouts 2 to 3 days each week.

Non-Impact Exercises
These movements don't immediately strengthen your bones. They can, nevertheless, increase your coordination and flexibility. That will lessen the likelihood that you'll fall and break a bone. You can do them every day.

Balance activities such as Tai Chi may improve your leg muscles and help you remain steadier on your feet. Posture exercises may help you battle against the "sloping" shoulders that might arise with osteoporosis and minimize your risk of spine fractures.

Routines such as yoga and Pilates help enhance strength, balance, and flexibility in patients with osteoporosis. But several of the actions you practice in these regimens — like forward-bending exercises — might make you more prone to acquire a fracture. If you're interested in these routines, consult with your doctor and ask your physical therapist to inform you of the safe movements and those you should avoid.

Exercise can help practically everyone with osteoporosis. But remember it's simply one aspect of a healthy treatment approach. Get lots of calcium and vitamin D in your diet, maintain a healthy weight, and don't smoke or drink too much alcohol. You also may require osteoporosis drugs to either grow or maintain your bone density. Work with your doctor to find out the best strategies to keep healthy and strong.

When Too Much Exercise Can Be Bad for Bones

Some data suggest that too much activity might contribute to bone issues, too. Intense exercise may induce hormone imbalances, which can lead to reduced bone mass, termed osteopenia. This may be a concern for some young female athletes. A mix of activity and recuperation is key to keeping osteoporosis at bay.

What To Add and What To Avoid

- The research indicated that smokers are at increased risk for muscles and weak bones than a non-smoker.
- Once the bone has thinned, it cannot be restored, it's possible to reduce the course of osteoporosis.
- The initial step in the therapy is to eradicate the source of osteoporosis if feasible. However, in women who have reached menopause therapy is geared at attempting to maintain the remaining bone, generally via Hormones Replacement Therapy (HRT).
- Most clinicians would agree that any woman who has early menopause (due to a hysterectomy, for example) or who has a family history of osteoporosis should be on (HRT).

- A high protein, calcium-rich diet, and frequent exercise assist to lessen the risk.